A Year of Living Sickishly:

A Patient Reflects

JESSIE GRUMAN

A YEAR OF LIVING SICKISHLY: A PATIENT REFLECTS

For more information: Health Behavior Media, Center for Advancing Health, 2000 Florida Avenue, N.W., Suite 210, Washington, D.C. 20009

Published by Health Behavior Media. Health Behavior Media books are published by the Center for Advancing Health.

Visit CFAH's website at www.cfah.org.

ISBN: 978-0-9815794-3-6

Serious illness is a group project. While the support of family, friends and colleagues has sustained me every step of the way, I have also been fortunate to work with clinicians who are smart, experienced and fluent in the current evidence in their fields. Each one of them invited me to join in planning my care and welcomed whatever participation I could muster during treatment as I swung back and forth between being too ill to speak and too curious to quit asking questions. I am grateful for their generosity, their wisdom, their flexibility and their care.

Table of Contents

Sick Suite

On September 27th, 2010, I had surgery to remove a cancerous tumor in my stomach. The following five essays describe some of my experiences during the next six weeks.

Reflections

Recovering from surgery, adjusting to life with a remodeled digestive system and chemotherapy shaped the subsequent year and provided opportunities for reflection.

Introduction

On Friday afternoon of Labor Day weekend three years ago, my doctor called to tell me that the pathology report from a recent endoscopy showed that I had stomach cancer. "Could you collect your husband and meet me in my office in an hour?"

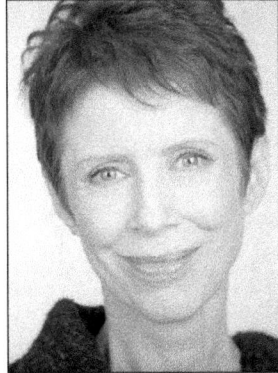

Maybe you can imagine what happened next.

At the time, I thought I could, since I had heard similar news three times before. But all my experience and all my expertise in health care did little to prepare me to meet the steep demands to find the right doctors and hospitals, choose the best treatments and then coordinate and participate fully in my care in the days following that phone call.

I am impressed by the advances in health care that made it possible to successfully (so far) treat this cancer. And I am deeply grateful to the clinicians and staff who worked with me every step of the way to plan and deliver that treatment. But I am also keenly aware of my own role in that success: how much I had to know and do to ensure that I would benefit from my health care.

Health care delivery is changing rapidly as technology advances and as health reform policies to reduce cost and improve quality and safety are implemented. But realizing the full potential of these changes rests on the often implicit assumption that we and our families knowledgeably and actively participate in our care.

The essays collected here reflect on what it felt like as a patient with a serious illness to do this: to cobble together a plan with my clinicians that works and to slog through the treatments in the hope that my cancer will be contained or cured and that I will be able to resume the interesting life I love.

Foreword

"Patient Engagement!" Our Skin Is in the Game

The idea that we should actively participate in our health care now attracts attention akin to the discovery of a cure for the common cold.

Here's how I learned about patient engagement:

On my 20th birthday, I was diagnosed with Hodgkin lymphoma and spent considerable time on life support while my doctors tried to halt the cancer's growth. I was devastated. I was just a child. I thought, "I can't die now — I'm just beginning!"

After I was well enough to go home, I began the daily trek to the hospital for weeks of radiation treatments, followed by two years of debilitating chemotherapy. I was skinny. I was hairless. And I was non-compliant.

Each time the doctor administered my chemotherapy, he would direct me to take six pills daily at regular intervals for the next two weeks. I didn't do it.

One day I might take two pills. Or six all at once. Some days I took none.

My doctor warned me to stay home because my immune system was at low ebb and I was at grave risk for infection.

I went out dancing.

I now look back at my behavior in awe and disbelief: Millions of dollars worth of biomedical research was distilled into the knowledge, experience, procedures and drugs aimed at a disease costing hundreds of thousands of dollars to treat. The impact of all this knowledge, experience, procedures and drugs ultimately largely relied on the actions of a weak, skinny, scared young person.

And I really struggled to make it work.

I was desperate not to die. But I couldn't follow my doctor's exact plan.

Why? Well, it was 1972, and there were no antiemetic drugs, which meant that I threw up every 15 minutes for 48 hours each week. My creative approach to pill taking was an attempt to find some brief respite from the physical torture — an hour of sleep, perhaps?

And I was young, deprived for months of friends and fun, longing for a sign that I might someday enjoy a normal life. How could a few hours of dancing hurt me if I was careful?

I was engaged in my health care — no doubt about it. I spent hours scheduling tests, sitting in waiting rooms, finding new specialists, filling prescriptions, ferrying records from doctor to doctor, urging them to communicate with one another, and receiving treatments. But sometimes short-term needs crowded out the long-term rewards of strict compliance with my treatment.

I marvel at the energy and effort I have devoted during my three subsequent cancer diagnoses to organize my care and follow the recommendations of my small army of doctors. And I am amazed that despite my knowledge, experience, confidence and commitment, I can still fall so short of doing what is recommended to save my own life.

The lesson that I take from my experience as an engaged, serial non-complier — and that I have learned from the hundreds of people I have interviewed about their experience with health care and illness — is that engagement in our care means we are trying over time to make the best possible use of health care services and technologies available to us.

This means that sometimes we have the wisdom, ease and discipline to take the long view: We exercise, eat modestly and keep tight control of our blood sugar now because we know it will benefit our health over time. Sometimes, immediate stresses crowd out our good intentions: We delay getting the colonoscopy because it eats up a whole day, and our jobs are already on the line. We choose to buy groceries rather than this month's supply of blood pressure medication.

A few health care leaders understand that engagement does not start and end with adherence to treatment. Judy Hibbard's Patient Activation Measure encourages professionals to plan interventions based on an assessment of our overall confidence in participating in preventing and treating disease.[1,2] Kate Lorig's Chronic Disease Self-Management Program gathers peer support and advice to help those with chronic conditions do the full range of tasks required to care for themselves.[3,4] Victor Montori and his group at the Mayo Clinic conduct research on "minimally disruptive" medicine.[5,6] David Sobel at the Permanente Medical Group develops programs and trains staff to help patients integrate the demands of their treatment into their busy lives.[7,8]

But this expansive understanding of engagement is far from the norm.

Growing recognition of patients' vital and considerable role in their health care is being sparked by new policies that link payment for services to outcomes and patients' experiences: pay for performance and other incentive programs for primary care clinicians, shared savings via accountable care organizations, Medicare payment policies to prevent re-hospitalizations, and patient experience-of-care ratings. Each of these nudges clinicians and institutions to set in place practices and policies that will reward them to help us participate more actively in our care.

Nonetheless, I have two persistent concerns about the way many professional stakeholders currently address patient engagement.

First, that programs to engage patients (or employees or members) in their health care target only very specific behaviors: Lose weight. Be physically active. Control blood sugar. Fill in the health risk appraisal.

And second, that engagement is most often equated with compliance. Increasingly, we must do these behaviors or we will be fired by our primary care doctor or will pay extra for health benefits.[9]

Engagement does not mean that we comply exactly with specific directives. Rather, it means that we act to the best of our ability to find and make good use of the health care available to us. The range of actions that we must take to benefit from our care far exceeds those few targeted behaviors:

- We must find the right doctors to care for us, consult with them, coordinate communication among them (in the absence of transportable electronic health records) and pay for their services.

- We must, with our clinicians' help, make informed decisions about care, participate in developing treatment plans and then implement our part of those plans over time.

- We must educate ourselves and act judiciously on what we learn about prevention, care for minor illnesses and attend to signs that indicate that any further delay in seeking care is dangerous.

Being engaged in our health care means trying to do all of this. Indeed, each of us must do all these things at some point if we are to realize the benefits of our health care. And we must do so even though we may be ill or frail or lack skills, knowledge, confidence or support.

We will not always be able to keep our eyes on the prize as defined by our clinicians. But we can be greatly helped by discussing our goals for treatment, knowing what our options are, what they cost in terms of time and money, and how they may affect our ability to work and play.

We often lack this information. Sometimes we need skills training to manage our symptoms and use our drugs and devices safely. All of us do better working with trusted, knowledgeable clinicians who help us set priorities and problem solve with us about how to care for ourselves and those we love.

I am alive today because I have been engaged in my health care. Without my efforts, all that beautiful science, all those marvelous innovations — the surgeries, the drugs, the devices — all my clinicians' experience and advice would have no effect. I have to do the best I can to show up, get the tests, eat as directed, take the pills, follow the advice and coordinate my care or I will not realize the benefit.

Trust me; our skin is already in the game.

SICK SUITE

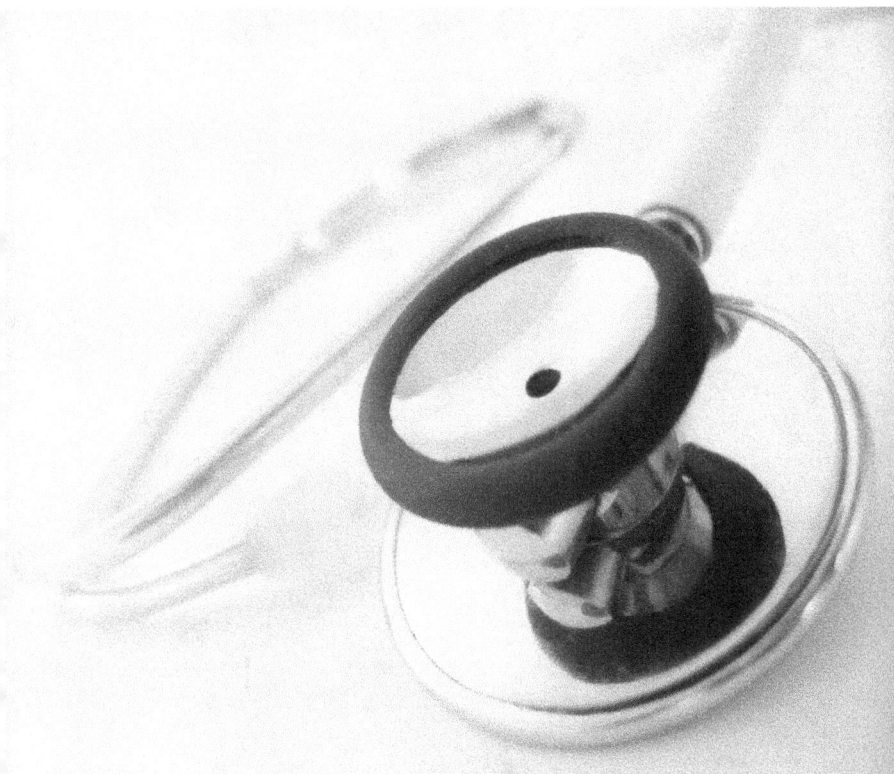

Another Devastating Diagnosis to Face

have stomach cancer and will undergo surgery today to remove part or all of my stomach.

While a truly expert writer would have documented the facts and his perceptions from the moment of discovery, I have been preoccupied with absorbing the shock, weighing my options and managing the logistics. I have been short on insight, long on anxiety.

But I have regained some composure since finalizing the plan for my immediate future, so I thought I'd try to capture some of my observations about this wild period this time around. After all, I listen all the time to people talk about how they experience these few weeks between a serious diagnosis and the beginning of treatment and, having gone through it repeatedly myself, I have a lot to compare it to.

A little background: This is my fourth cancer-related diagnosis. My stomach cancer was discovered due to the vigilance of my primary care doctor who treats adult survivors of childhood cancer and who leaves no symptom — regardless of how seemingly minor — unexplored. I had dismissed my insignificant symptom once it disappeared after a few days. However, my doctor didn't, and it turned out to be a small gastric tumor, probably a result of the high doses of radiation that were the standard of treatment for my stage of Hodgkin's disease in the early 1970s. The tumor will be removed, along with as much of my stomach as is necessary to prevent its recurrence. While the size of the tumor and its staging leave me optimistic that I won't need chemotherapy and radiation, I won't know for certain until a week after surgery.

Here are some of my thoughts that have been swirling around:

Are you kidding? *Again?* I was just starting to feel like maybe I'm normal — not a perpetual cancer patient. This is so disruptive for me, for my beloved family, colleagues and friends! I'm worried by how long it is taking to set up my plan: Is the cancer spreading while I'm auditioning surgeons? I'm struggling to hold onto my belief in randomness, trying to not blame myself for doing something that caused this. Every hour, this situation looks different: Just when I start feeling optimistic, my imagination coughs up a new horrific scenario.

Breaking through this turmoil are bright flashes of gratitude: for the amazing luck of finding the tumor while it is small; for my access to smart doctors who take me seriously and who will do their best for me; for my intense, indefatigable, funny husband; for my brother Pete, who has left his family to entertain (distract) us during these few days; for my family, my friends and colleagues who offer words of support and gestures of solidarity.

I remain impressed by the number of life-changing choices I must make quickly to respond to a serious diagnosis. You may know that I wrote a book about how to maneuver through this period after my last serious diagnosis, for which I interviewed more than 200 people, including many experts.[1] Well, I went back and re-read the book last week. It provides good guidance. But despite listening to all those stories and carefully laying out the logic for why and how to respond, despite all my expertise in using scientific evidence to make health care choices, and despite all my experience responding to my different diagnoses, I still don't seem to be able to coldly examine the facts and evaluate the surgeon's strategy as though I were choosing which laptop to buy. "Doing the best I can" is probably a more realistic description of how I'm able to approach this, rather than being a "savvy health care consumer."

I have a newfound understanding of the gravity of shared decision making. When my surgeon tells me about the risks associated with the different possible approaches to surgery and asks my preference, she implicitly is asking me to assume the risks of the choice I make. I am reluctant to respond, not sure I know enough to choose. If I get it wrong and the outcome is bad, will it be my own fault? But at the same time, it is inconceivable to me that she would make this decision — which certainly will have an impact on the quality, if not the length, of my life — without me.

And I'm realizing that at the end of the day, it doesn't matter how much I know or what I believe or how ready I think I am to die. It doesn't matter what books I've read or what books I've written: The news of a serious cancer diagnosis packs a powerful punch. And that punch affects not only me. It produces a wave of distress that washes in various ways over my family, friends, co-workers and acquaintances.

One lesson I've learned from my previous experiences, however, is that within a few weeks the wave will abate. We'll all calm down. And with some idea of what lies ahead, my family and I will adapt to the new demands of my treatment one step at a time while I assemble a version of the life I had before.

Right now, however, the first episode of my current illness is ending. I'm making the last few phone calls and straightening my desk. This morning I will become a patient: I'll turn the responsibility for my future over to those whose skills, expertise and compassion can make their unique contribution to my ongoing effort to live as well as I can for as long as I can.

I'll let you know how it goes.

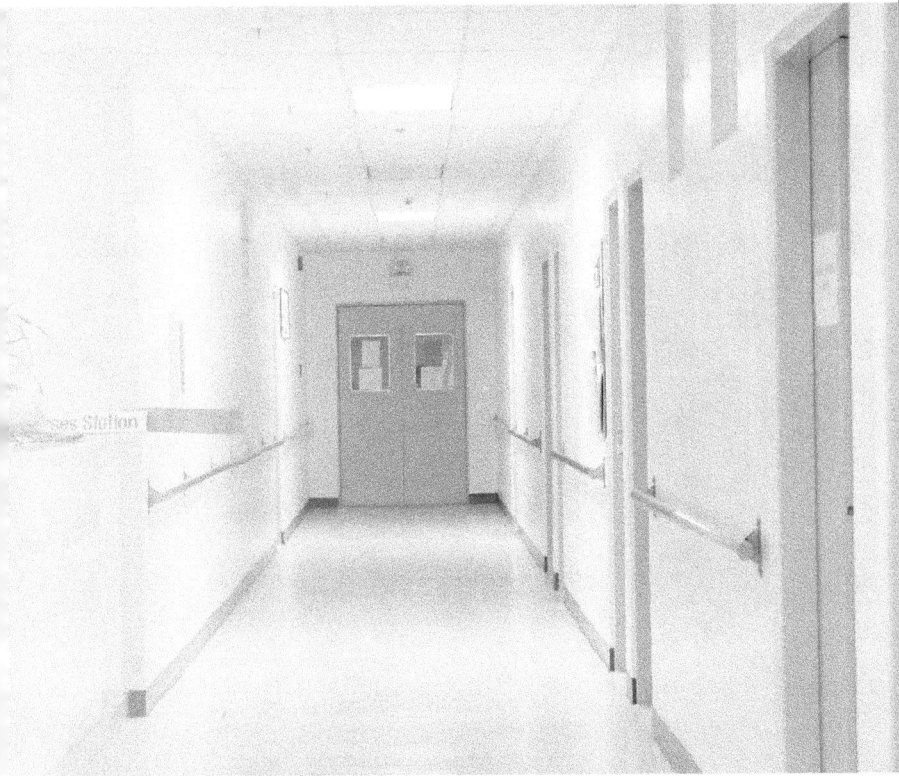

Patient Engagement on the Med-Surg Floor

Three times a day, as though responding to some signal audible only to the generously medicated, we rise from our beds to join the slow procession around the perimeter of the unit. Like slumped, disheveled royalty, each of us blearily leads our retinue of anxious loved ones who push our IV poles, bear sweaters to ward off the harsh air conditioning and hover to prevent stumbles. Some make eye contact. Few talk. Each of us is absorbed in our suffering and our longing to return to bed.

This is one glimpse of what it means to be engaged in our health care. I find the experience strangely moving.

Despite the nausea, dizziness and enough mind-altering drugs to fell a horse, so many of us fight our way to consciousness, creakily right ourselves and step out of our rooms to join the others. At that moment we are able to say, "I'll do the one thing they say might help me get better," taking one painstaking step after the next — the height of our ambition meets the limits of our abilities — to resume the life we left behind when we entered the hospital.

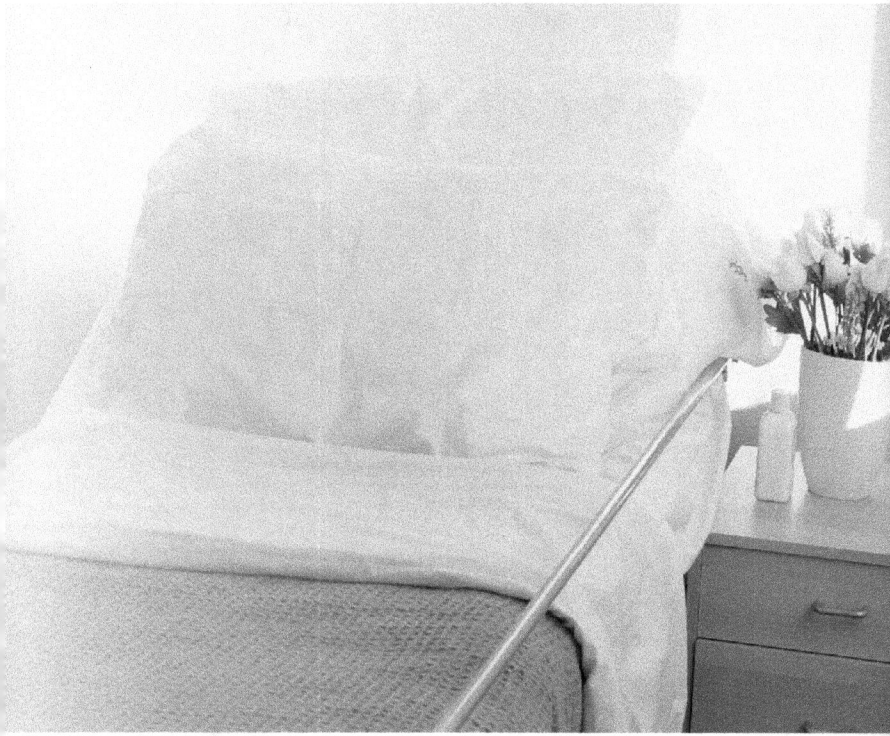

Contemplating Safety While Lying Down

"**Y**ou have to get out of this hospital — it's a dangerous place," each of my physician friends exclaimed when they came to visit me during my recent stay after surgery for stomach cancer.

Jeez! I *know!* Prior to my operation, I was more preoccupied with the possibility of medical errors than with the operation itself or the pain it might cause. What if they take out my kidney instead of my stomach? Or leave a sponge in there? Or over-hydrate me so I drown? What if one of my many overnight vitals-taking-shot-givers exposes me to a staph infection or infects me with MRSA?

The human imagination has wondrous capacities, especially when fueled by true stories of harm that people have experienced due to medical errors. I read closely the Institute of Medicine report, *To Err Is Human: Building a Safer Health System;* I am horrified by the medical errors experienced by Susan Sheridan and impressed by her leadership of Consumers Advancing Patient Safety and by Diane Pinakiewicz's efforts at the National Patient Safety Foundation to raise awareness about the dangers patients face due to carelessness and lack of system-level controls.[1-4]

But for all my well-informed apprehension and the warnings of danger by my doctor friends during my recent hospital stay, I was in no condition to be vigilant about my care. I was far too ill. Not too ill to forget the danger, especially when repeatedly reminded of it, but too befuddled by the after-effects of anesthesia and the pain medication to actually track the actions of the many health professionals who poked at me day and night. My husband, a constant presence during the day, was hyper-alert, but often I was on my own: in the operating room, during the hours spent getting various scans, and overnight.

And so I spent those seven days on tenterhooks, worried about the dangers that lurked in and on the hands of each doctor, friendly nurse and aide.

What is the real aim of efforts to inform the public about medical errors and the appalling state of patient safety in U.S. hospitals?

Is it to get us to choose the hospital we use based on hospital performance reports? That is an optimistic goal to date.[5] The primary impact of those ratings appears to be to prompt hospitals to improve specific clinical services that are rated, not to shape patient choices among different institutions.

Are these public education efforts an attempt to spark a citizen uprising against medical errors? Hmm. If the current public climate is any indication, competition for our outrage is pretty stiff and most of us are more focused on putting our hospital experience — especially if it is negative — behind us.

Is the aim to ensure that we are vigilant while we are in the hospital? Yes, our loved ones should watch out for us while we are hospitalized, although many of us don't have the person-power in our lives to mount a 24-hour watch. However, as a patient whose husband was mostly there but sometimes was not, I was frightened by the messages about the possibility of harm caused by my care. They permeated my dreams and contributed to an anxious wariness about each staff person who entered my room.

Would I rather not know about the risks of medical errors? Not for a moment. If there is a danger, I want to protect myself as well as I can. I strongly support the work of dedicated volunteers across the country to educate us about those risks.

But I am also acutely aware of this shift in responsibility, this additional task that patients and families must take on to ensure that we benefit from our care. And I am concerned that this is yet another example of how, in the name of "choice," "patient-centeredness" and "autonomy," we are carefully informed about the risks of our health care while most of us actually possess little of the experience, judgment or ability to act effectively to reduce them.

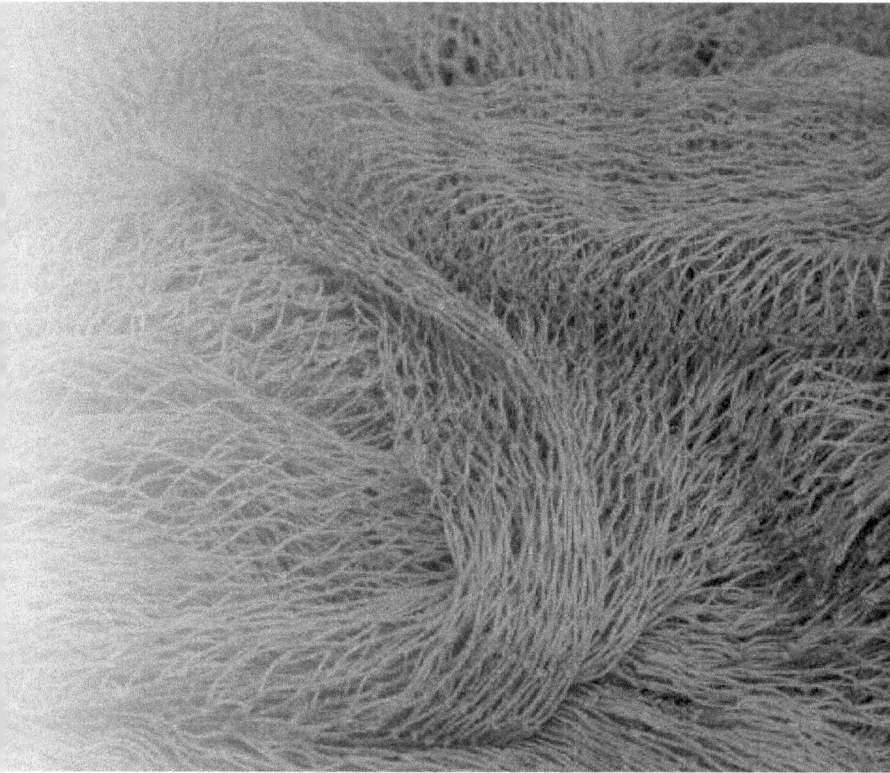

Hospital Discharge Without a Net

By the time I reached the sixth day of my hospitalization for stomach cancer surgery, I was antsy to go home and I quizzed each nurse and physician who came into my room about what must happen for me to be liberated the following day. Their responses were consistent: My surgeon would visit in the morning and write orders for my release. Then I would have a comprehensive discussion with my nurse about my discharge plan, after which I could leave.

I was pretty curious about getting that discharge plan. The Patient Protection and Affordable Care Act raised the stakes for hospitals to reduce high readmission rates, and new data on those rates are now available.[1,2] The rates and approaches to reduce them through improved discharge planning are the subject of news reports, journal articles and conferences.[3-7] And I, a patient in a modern, quality-conscious hospital, was going to experience this process myself!

Here's a rough transcript of my discharge discussion which began at 8:43 a.m.:

Nurse: Good news! The orders came through! You can go home.

Me: (In the corner untangling wires from my cellphone and iPod chargers) Wonderful. What do I need to know?

Nurse: Here are a couple prescriptions for pain medication. Don't drive if you take it. Call your surgeon if you have a temperature or are worried about anything. Go see your doctor in two weeks. Do you want a flu shot? I can give you one before you leave. If you need a wheelchair to take you to the door, I'll call for one. If not, you can go home. Take care of yourself. You are going to do *great*!

That was it: 8:45 a.m., and I could leave.

Now, I am a sucker for encouraging words, but right then, I wasn't sure I knew how to operate my new digestive system, plus my midsection looked like a gutted fish. Could I injure myself? What should I do to prevent complications or pain? After all, until this moment every milliliter of input and output to and from my body was measured, every perturbation in temperature, blood pressure and blood sugar was scrutinized every few hours and swiftly responded to with drugs or tests. Did I now need to assume this level of vigilance in order to be safe?

"Use your judgment. Take it easy. You'll do fine."

Fortunately, my nurse was right. I have taken it easy. I have used whatever judgment I could scrape together between naps to guide my eating and physical activity. And I am slowly regaining my energy.

However, this brief discussion didn't prepare me for the transition from complete dependence to complete independence. It did not allow me to leave the hospital confident that I could care for myself. And it would have done nothing to help mobilize patients and families who are less aware than I am of the many demands of post-surgical care at home.

I know that my nurse delivered my discharge plan as required: I have the paper she read from in front of me now. And I know that, as part of the hospital quality rating effort, she checked off the box in my record indicating that she had done so. But I wanted more: I wanted details about what might go wrong, when to worry and which small changes to ignore. I wanted to know what I had to do to help myself get better. I wanted to know how much and what kind of help I would need to care for myself. *I wanted some acknowledgement of the gravity of what I had just experienced and the magnitude of the responsibility that was now mine.*

Would it make any difference to my current health status if had I received what I wanted? I don't know. Scant research has been conducted on this specific question. Would it have helped me and my husband prepare to take over my care? Yes.

And here is the curious point where the *impulse* to deliver health care that is supportive of our engagement in our care bumps into the *reality* of the strategies available to actually make such changes: Vital interpersonal interactions between professionals and patients too easily collapse into thoughtless, routine check-the-box exercises when they become required by institutional performance measures.[8] Inquiries about completed advance directives and pharmacy counseling are other examples of where this happens.[9,10]

The Centers for Medicare and Medicaid Services has a well-established requirement for patient hospital discharge planning that reflects the common-sense idea that we do better when we have the knowledge and skills to care for ourselves when we are discharged from the hospital.[11] The need to ensure that we are able to do so has only become more urgent as advances in technology make it possible for us to return home quicker yet sicker, taking on the tasks of medication, diet and rehabilitation previously performed by professionals.[12]

But it's going to take a lot more than a 90-second discharge discussion to help us perform these tasks as well as we can. There are some well-designed approaches that have the potential to make a difference, but their effectiveness depends not only on resources, but also on institutional and professional commitment.[13-15] What will spark widespread, sustained implementation of such comprehensive discharge programs that will ensure that all of us can competently care for ourselves and our loved ones after a hospital stay?

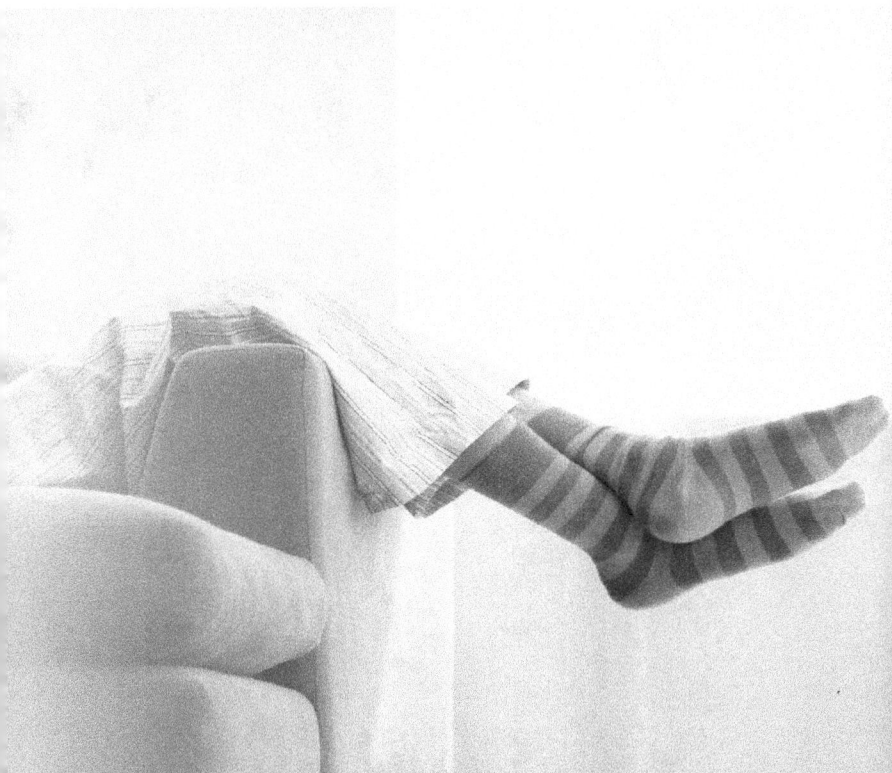

5

Friends, Fatigue and the Slow Slog Back

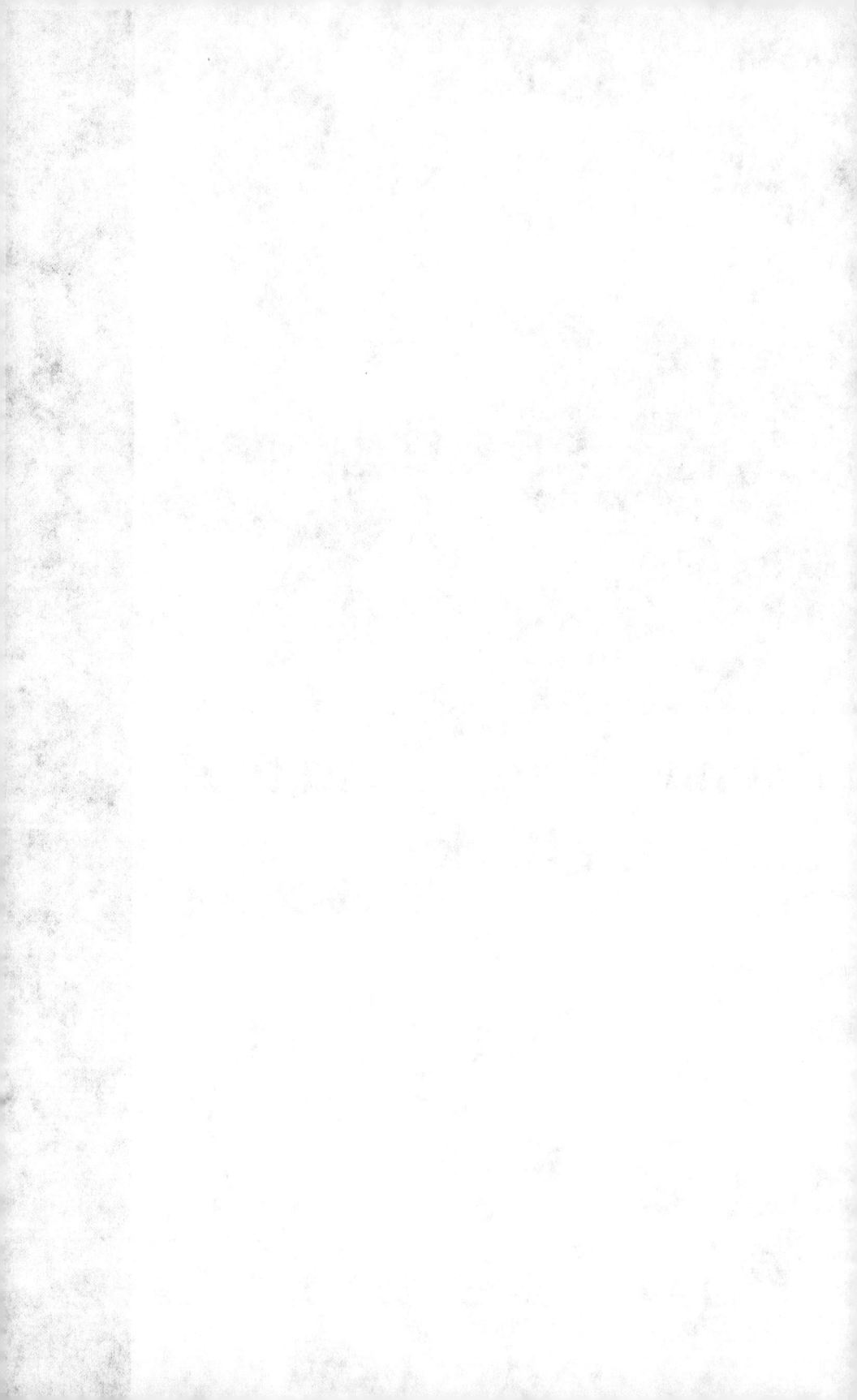

have much experience with serious illness. And so I am a connoisseur of fatigue: the sleepless edginess of post-radiation fatigue, the heavy constancy of cardiac fatigue, the blur and blues of chemotherapy-related fatigue.

I am learning again about post-surgical fatigue, which this time is characterized by short bursts of energy randomly emerging from an otherwise constant, whacked-upside-the-head-with-a-golf-club, sleeping and waking fog.

Regardless of the flavor, it is the force of fatigue that exacerbates the discomforts and symptoms of an illness. It is fatigue that makes each sip of water an action to be carefully planned, each trip to the refrigerator an accomplishment. It is fatigue that exhausts my hands holding a book and my mind when reading more than a few sentences. It is fatigue that shrinks my world to the size of my living room, leaching the meaning from family news, work developments and the impending election.

Fatigue diminishes me: I consist of only this disease, this body.

Into this gray desolation drop brief messages of support, of encouragement, of good wishes. These words are not sent to the thin figure lying on the couch staring at the sky. Rather, they are addressed to a friend, acquaintance, colleague, daughter or sister — a person, who stands up straight, is passionately engaged in her life and has a lot of work to do.

These messages remind me of the parts of myself that are eclipsed by my illness. And they reassure me that I will be able to find those parts again.

I am grateful for each one.

REFLECTIONS

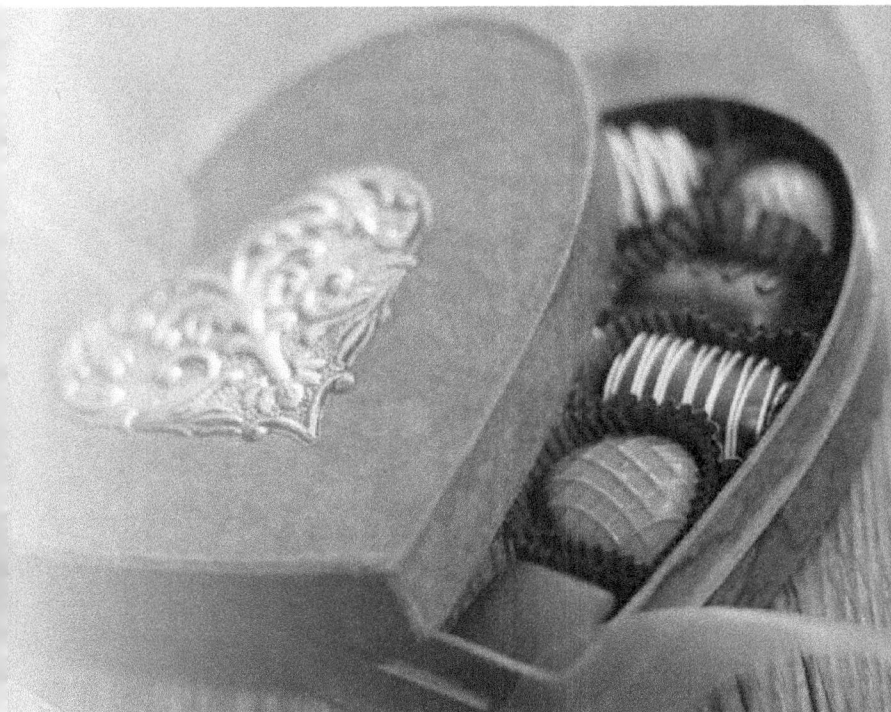

6

A Valentine to Shared Decision Making

S hared decision making is hot right now. Research.[1] Surveys. Tools.[2] Training. Conferences.[3] Policies.

The current model of shared decision making consists of providing patients with evidence that allows them to compare the risks and side effects of different treatments or preventive services when more than one option is available.[4] After studying the evidence, the theory goes, patients discuss it with their physician, weigh their personal preferences and together agree upon a course of action.

As an advocate for policies that support people's engagement in their health care and a veteran of a few serious illnesses, I support this approach. But I have also been a cancer patient and have found it hard to align the neatness of shared decision making that exists in the warm environment of the conference room with the cold reality of the exam room. It seems idealized, isolated from the clutter of health care delivery and the emotional and physical ebb and flow of illness. As a professional, I looked forward to an orderly process of sharing decisions with my oncologist. Here is my week-to-week experience, not much different than that of the average patient:

Week 1: I meet my oncologist. I had surgery a few weeks before to remove a tumor in my stomach. I am still foggy with fatigue, but I've poked around online to learn about possible treatments. He describes the current evidence about the disease and its treatment. I tell him I'm worried that the chemotherapy will make it hard to think and write. We decide to finalize a plan at my next visit once I have regained some strength.

Week 3: I feel better. I've consulted a number of oncologists to get their treatment recommendations and I've read more studies, some recommended by my oncologist. He answers my many questions about the evidence and the other opinions. We look together at survival curves for patients with my cancer at this stage and commiserate about the lack of evidence about which mix of drugs might lead to the best result. After talking for an hour, we agree on a chemotherapy regimen to start two days later.

Week 4: I struggle hard to concentrate during the visit, but my thinking is blurred. I haven't eaten or drunk much for days because of the nausea caused by the chemotherapy. I want to know how to reduce the side effects of the chemotherapeutic agents and the drugs used to counteract the side effects.

Week 5: I have almost no recollection of this meeting. I feel so sick I can barely sit up. I give monosyllabic answers to my oncologist's questions. Before he bundles me off to be rehydrated, we decide to stop the treatment.

How many important decisions did we make together about my care over these few weeks? How many of them were preference-sensitive? How many involved a formal display of evidence? And in how many of those decisions was I a rational, informed participant?

Those who work to enable individuals to engage more fully in their care (and professionally, I include myself here) concentrate their efforts in a space that lies somewhere between a rock and a hard place. The "rock" is the fact that most of us are mostly well most of the time and so have little interest in learning about the range of diseases that we might someday contract or the treatments we may someday need. The "hard place" is illustrated above: When we are faced with health care decisions, many of us are frightened or our minds are clouded by pain.

Shared decision making assumes that a generous zone of calm and clarity lies between that rock and that hard place; that health decisions are made when our willingness to pay attention coincides with our ability to find relevant, unbiased information, weigh it against our preferences and make sound judgments about our care, unhindered by our suffering and in collaboration with a trusted health care provider.

For some decisions — get a PSA test? have surgery for heel pain? — this zone may exist. But anxiety and suffering can interfere with rational deliberation for even minor decisions. When we are ill, the likelihood of interference is even greater.

Why, then, is so much activity directed toward this sweet moment of converging sanity, capacity and data?

A while ago I attended (via the Web) a conference convened by the leading voice in this field, the Informed Medical Decisions Foundation.[5] After listening to the speakers at the conference, this is my answer:

Because we need a good model.

It is important to have and promote a step-by-step process to present us and our families with evidence that helps us understand the trade-offs of health decisions and to thus prepare for productive discussions with our physicians. And it is important to know that most individuals and physicians who go through this formal process find it feasible and satisfying.

But it is the values that this model embodies that justify the focus, energy and investments in it. These values are that:

- Information and evidence about tests and treatments are *critical components* of many health care decisions.

- Patients and caregivers can *understand evidence and use it* to help them weigh their options.

- Providers can *discuss available evidence* — what is known, where it is lacking and what it means — with patients.

- Patients are explicitly *invited to participate* in decisions about their care (even if that participation consists of delegating decision making to a caregiver or physician).

- The *opinions and preferences* of patients — informed by their understanding of the evidence — shape and determine the tests they take and the treatment they undergo.

For most Americans, these values are not reflected in current expectations about their role in their care. Nor do these values shape the day-to-day practices of most providers.

Shared decision making is an aspirational model that delineates changes that are necessary, given the increasing number of options we face in making good use of our health care. In its precision, the model demonstrates to us, our caregivers and our providers just how these values might guide the many decisions that we navigate together every day.

Sure, the choice before me, my abilities and my condition will always influence the way my physician and I interact. And of course, the progression of science will by its nature limit the depth and breadth of any formal set of evidence I review.

But the values embedded in shared decision making were woven through the five weeks I describe here, even when my doctor and I were in "hard places." My participation in my care was enabled and expected. My choices guided my treatment. My provider and I worked together to ease my suffering.

The importance now accorded to shared decision making is driving a shift in the values and behavior of us all.

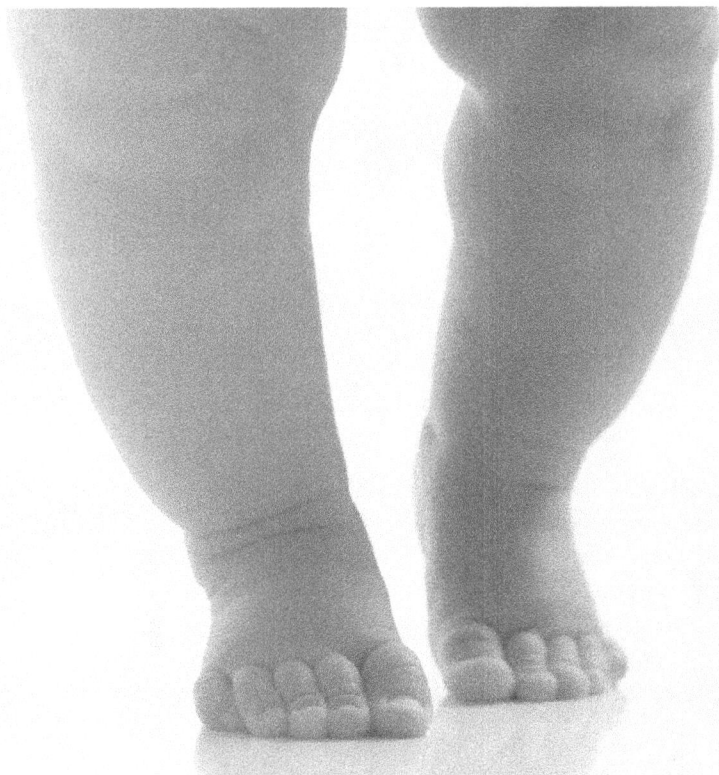

One Small Step for Patient-Centered Care, One Less Barrier to Engagement

As far as my chemo nurse Olga* is concerned, I can do nothing right.

She scolded me for sending an email when she thought I should have called and vice versa. She scolded me for going home before my next appointment was scheduled. She scolded me for asking to speak to her personally instead of whichever nurse was available. She scolded me for calling my oncologist directly. She scolded me for asking whether my clinical information and questions are shared between my oncologist and the staff of the chemo suite. I could go on...

"Funny," I think to myself. "If she had told me the basic ground rules of interacting with her and her colleagues, I would have been happy to follow them. Otherwise, how am I supposed to know — guess?"

While my diagnosis of stomach cancer in the fall of 2010 introduced me to many new doctors and their practices, most were one-shot consultations. Other than making sure the test results they ordered and their recommendations found their way to the right physicians (my responsibility in the absence of an interoperable health record), it didn't really matter how I communicated with them over time.

But when you start chemotherapy or have a heart attack, brain injury, stroke or a serious chronic condition, you sign on to a long-term relationship with a whole crew of people — receptionists, various types of nurses, aides, physical therapists, educators, coaches, phlebotomists, pharmacists and doctors — that is likely to require a lot of back-and-forth. Chances are that these professionals have figured out ways to work together pretty efficiently. The problem is that most of them don't let us in on the action; they rarely provide us with (ahem) "rules of engagement" that would tell us how to work most effectively with them.

And so we are left to guess. And when we guess wrong, we risk being scolded. This, of course, leaves us frustrated...sometimes even mildly rebellious.

In interviews that the Center for Advancing Health (CFAH) conducted about receiving care after a serious diagnosis, patients and families raised their bewilderment (and annoyance) about the difficulty of learning how to communicate with their specialists. The same was heard from people discussing their regular providers. People can't figure out how to get their test results. They are puzzled about who to call after hours or on weekends. They are baffled about who they should talk to regarding billing and insurance problems. They are flummoxed by the new and unfamiliar demands placed on them by different sources of continuing care: rehabilitation hospitals, cardiac rehab, oncology suites, neurologists and other specialists, and for some, unfamiliar primary care medical homes.[1]

The confusion of patients and families will not in itself drive any widespread change in the way care is delivered. But our endless stream of identical questions to busy professionals surely interferes with their efficiency. And with increasing calls for the competent engagement of patients and families, making explicit the ways we can most effectively work with a team of professionals seems like a modest, feasible step for primary and specialty care providers to take. Doing so is one aspect of making our care truly patient- and family-centered that doesn't require access to a high-tech solution or federal policy nudge.[2,3]

So consider, then: A couple years ago, in response to interview findings, CFAH developed, with Susan Edgman-Levitan and her colleagues at Massachusetts General Hospital, a model guide for patients and caregivers that identified the basic information people need to interact over time with a given medical practice or setting.[4] The model includes items such as: 1) the names of the care team members; 2) a description of who is responsible for responding to which concerns; for instance, questions about symptoms, appointments, insurance and phone numbers; 3) how to get prescription refills; 4) procedures for after-hours and emergency care; 5) access to health records; 6) the process for reporting on tests; and even 7) information about parking and public transportation.

Recently, a group of primary care practices decided they would pilot test this model. Weeks later they abandoned the effort. Why? Because the clinicians within the practices couldn't agree on their office hours.

Sigh.

Not her real name.

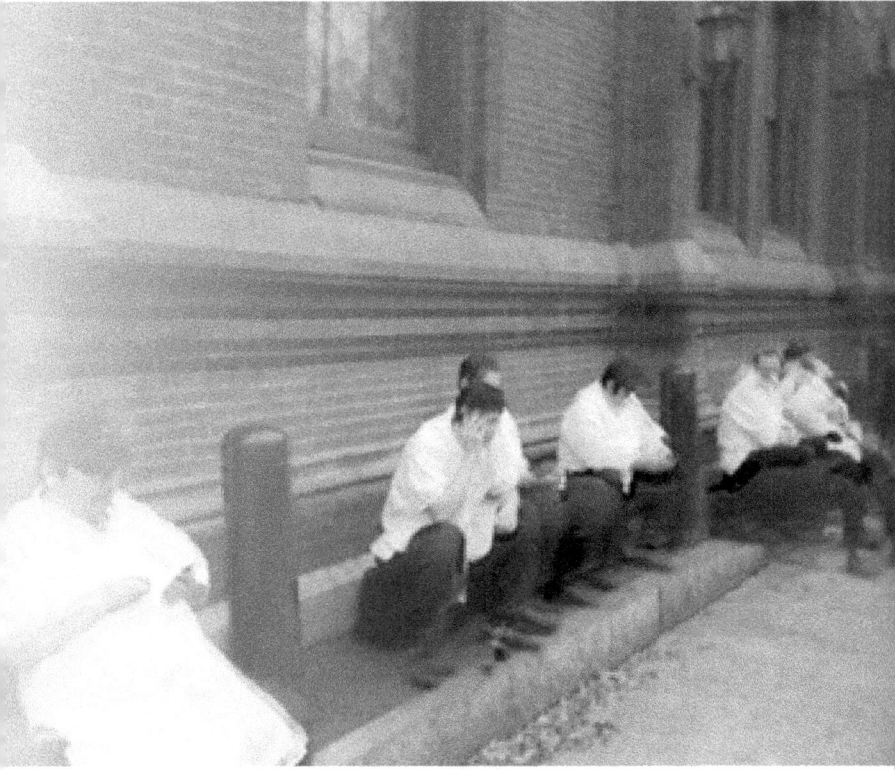

I Am Not My iPhone

There is excitement in the air about how mobile phones are the breakthrough technology for changing health behavior. Last Saturday, I was convinced this must be true. In two short hours, I:

- Skimmed the *New York Times* op-ed, *You Love Your iPhone. Literally*, which (questionably) claimed that functional MRIs show that our brains react to our iPhones the same way they do to the proximity of someone we love.[1,2]

- Received an email on my iPhone from NYC Health Business Leaders inviting me to come to a meeting: *Is Mobile Health the Next Killer App?*[3]

- Came across a podcast on how mobile technology is going to vastly change care for seniors with chronic conditions.[4]

- Read a beautiful review of the behavior change literature that asks the question: *Is Mobile the Prescription for Sustained Behavior Change?*[5]

- Received a text about the highly anticipated release of the iPhone 5.

- Came across the entire kitchen crew of a fancy restaurant staring into or talking on their mobile phones.

Now I'm sure that the seductive power of mobile phones hasn't escaped your notice. Certainly, if you are concerned about people engaging more fully in their health and health care, you have seen the thousands of apps that intend to exploit the combination of widely available mobile phones with advances in Web-enabled technology as the new best way to spark and sustain health behavior change.

I love the optimism that has driven the development of these apps to date. The theoretical reasoning of behavioral scientists that finds mobile apps to be a potential game changer is subtle and compelling — this is why this technology is different and what it offers above all other technologies and approaches. And I love imagining the personalized guidance and support that will be available to us once these theories are transformed into more sophisticated apps for our mobile devices.

I also love it because this health and lifestyle behavior change stuff is really hard for us — whether we are individuals or caregivers or clinicians — and it is really important. It's necessary for many of us to act differently if we are going to become or remain active and healthy.

We love our phones. They distract us when we are lonely or bored and inform us when we are lost or curious. They allow us freedom of place and space. And the rewards they offer are immediate, efficient and entertaining. But we mostly love them because we like what they do for us.

My friend Lou has early Alzheimer's disease, and her caregivers have set up a locator app on her iPhone to track her when she goes out. When her resentment about being spied on builds up, she hides her phone in her house and heads for the door, almost always forgetting where she put it or that she hid it at all. Even in her confused state, she's willing to let go of that treasured phone — which is her main link to the people she loves — when she associates it with negative emotions and experiences.

I am trying to gain weight. I want to eat and know I should eat every hour and I have a full array of tempting snacks by my side at all times. And I have carefully set up an app to deliver a different alarm every hour to prompt me to eat. Yet I reliably delay my response to each alarm and then forget to eat the nuts and even the cookies. You cannot imagine how easy it is to turn that little sucker off and promise myself that I'll eat as soon as the conference call is over, when I finish this paragraph, or when I get off the subway.

Two small examples, but telling ones.

While mobile phones can do so much and will soon be able to do much more — monitor our movements, tailor information to our interests, send us strategic messages, and remind us with alarms — our will is still our own. When the device, rather than us, becomes the driver of change, it becomes an electronic substitute for a nagging parent or spouse, a voice that reins in and confines, bringing out our worst adolescent tendencies: mischief, defiance, disobedience. I'm not sure an app exists that can wrangle that impulse into submission in most of us most of the time.

We prefer fun, enjoyable activities and avoid irritating ones. If an app becomes the source of unwelcome advice or beeps or we feel intruded upon or our response to some app brings unwanted attention to us, we will have no problem circumventing it.

As much as we depend on the convenience of our mobile devices, they are only tools. While my mobile phone can link me to information, advice, friends and support, I don't confuse *it* with *them*. I can get to these valuable resources via my phone when I want them. But I know that when I am sick, the disease is located in my body, not my phone. Regardless of what is going on with my phone, I'm the one who has the cancer and I'm the one who takes the chemotherapy drugs, pleased as I would be to delegate that responsibility to an inanimate object. When the alarm goes off that my mom has fallen, it is my hands or the hands of the EMR technician that help her get up, not the mobile device. When Lou gets lost, even when she has her phone with her, it is her caregivers or the police who find her and bring her home.

I am convinced that behavioral scientists and app developers will be successful in getting those mobile phones to do what they want them to: deliver clever, tailored behavior change strategies directly to us. And I am equally confident that many of us will try those apps. But if they don't do what we want them to — if they become a burden, an intrusion or a bore — we will ignore them, delete them, or, when all else fails, carefully place our beloved phone in the vegetable drawer of the refrigerator and head out the door.

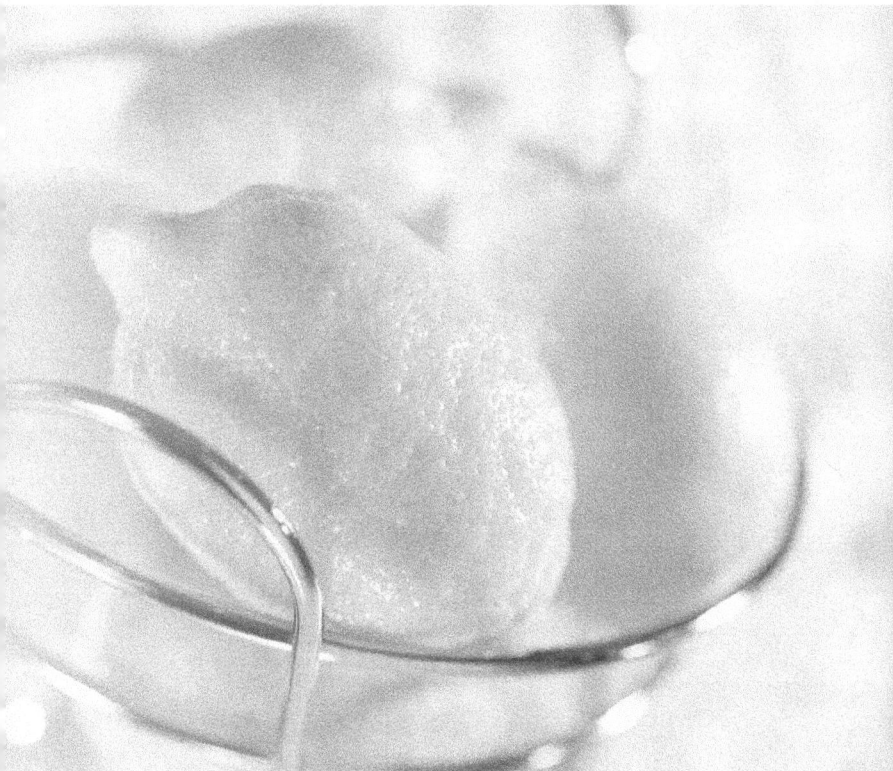

9

The Lemon of Illness and the Demand for Lemonade

"*Life gives you lemons and you make lemonade...your response to all those cancer diagnoses is so positive, such a contribution!" "Your work demonstrates that illness is a great teacher." "Your illness has been a blessing in disguise.*"

Well-meaning, thoughtful people have said things like this to me since I started writing about what I have to do to make my health care work for me when I am seriously ill. I generally hear in such comments polite appreciation of my efforts, which is nice because I know that people often struggle with what to say when confronted by others' hardships.

But beneath that appreciation I detect a common belief about the nature of suffering (from illness in particular) that in its inaccuracy can inadvertently hurt sick people and those who love them.

The belief is that sickness ennobles us, that there is good to be found in the experience of illness; while diseases are bad, they teach life lessons that are good.

The damage comes from the expectation — mine, my family's, my work colleagues', those of society at large — that I will seek and *find* meaning in my illness. That I will, as a consequence of my illness, become a wiser, better person. If I do not find spiritual or philosophical benefit, I fall short: Either I haven't tried hard enough or I'm not smart enough to do so.

It is tough when I am sick to accept the fragility of my own body. The chores of illness are unpleasant and combined with fatigue, pain and other symptoms, they absorb most of my energy. I am already doing the best I can to get better. To add to these challenges the expectation that the experience of illness will reorder my priorities and make me wiser (or gentler or kinder or more generous) burdens me further. Not only has my body failed, I might now also fail as a person.

The inaccuracy is that illness is no different from any other life event: Sometimes we learn from experience, sometimes we don't. Of course we can learn from bad times, just as we do from good ones. A car accident can result in piercing insight about what is truly valuable in life;

the death of a parent can spark life-altering reflections about time and the future.

Sweet are the uses of adversity,
Which like the toad, ugly and venomous,
Wears yet a jewel in his crown.
And this our life, exempt from public haunt,
Finds tongues in trees, books in running brooks,
Sermons in stone, and good in every thing.

In Shakespeare's *As You Like It*, Duke Senior makes this comment about the very human urge to make sense of nature and our penchant to find benefit in adversity.[1] Psychologists and anthropologists have long studied our tendency to construct explanations and find meaning in random events.[2,3] Indeed, the growing fields of narrative medicine and expressive writing recognize the value to patients of writing and telling — and physicians listening to — our explanations of the ebbs and flows in our health.[4,5]

But none of these approaches holds illness separate as an experience that uniquely confers benefit, as though meaning and wisdom are the bright side of the bad penny of illness, and that finding that bright side is the responsibility of the person who is sick.

Recent research purports to show that those who report finding a benefit from their illness do better — are less depressed, heal faster or live longer.[6] These studies presumably will lead to "interventions" to urge or teach those of us who are sick to search our souls for the spiritual and interpersonal benefits our suffering has brought us. Should we be reluctant or unable to do so means we have failed ourselves or our loved ones: We haven't been able to take this action that, even if it doesn't succeed in ameliorating our pain or extending our lives, might at least make us easier to live with while we are sick.

I write about what it takes to find and make good use of health care because I have spent so much time figuring out how to do it. I hope that my reflections can help others avoid some of my mistakes. I also write about the experience of illness to challenge the vision of patients' designated roles as energetic advocates for ourselves and for health system change as envisioned by media, government and health policy experts. We have experienced a dramatic increase in the complex demands placed on us by a health care system that is uncoordinated and chaotic. If I, with my education, experience and privilege, struggle to meet these demands in order to benefit from the procedures, drugs, devices and services available to me when I am ill, what happens to people who know and have less than I do?

One could argue that in the adversity of four cancer-related diagnoses, a dangerous heart condition and all of the treatments they entail, I have found the calling and the commitment to speak out on behalf of people who are ill. Maybe. But this is neither a sign of my virtue nor of my will. I would trade that commitment in one hot second to not have been sick in the first place.

My writing about illness may be a jewel in the crown of a toad. But all that illness? Not lemonade. Not a lesson. Not a blessing.

Just a toad.

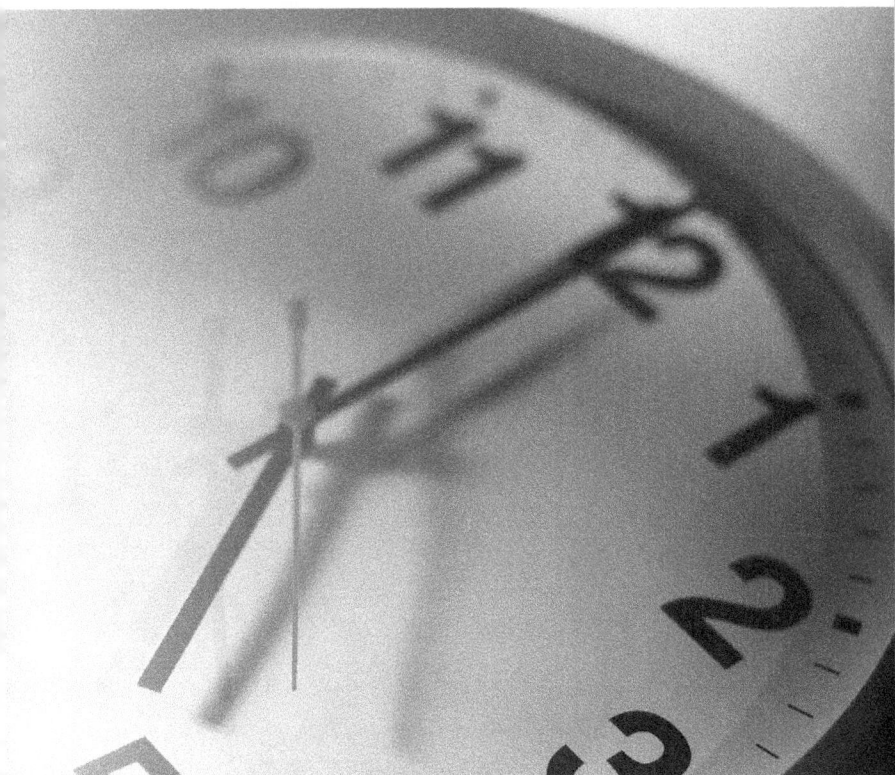

10

Appointment in Samarra: Our Lives of Watchful Waiting

Watchful waiting has become a way of life for many of us.

Last week, Sam had his first six-month scan following treatment for esophageal cancer. It showed that the original cancer had not recurred and that the tumors behind his eyes and the hot spots on his kidneys and liver hadn't grown. Sam and his wife, Sonia, are celebrating for a few days before they return to worrying, checking for symptoms and counting the days until the next scan.

The sound technician for my talk in Chicago this week recounted how 17 years after his radical prostatectomy, he insists on having his PSA tested every six months, despite the one-year interval recommended by the guideline. "From the time the blood is drawn to when I get the results, I'm still a wreck. And in between tests, my worry is like a pebble in my shoe...it's small, but it's always there."

Usually we think of watchful waiting as a strategy recommended to people who have a condition that may or may not develop into something requiring medical intervention: a consistently elevated PSA, persistent debilitating back pain, an arthritic hip.[1] The problem is checked by our doctor periodically to see if it is progressing and at what rate, with the intent of starting treatment only if and when the problem is clearly a threat or significantly erodes our quality of life.

However, this identical medical strategy is used widely to treat a growing number of people who also wait watchfully, although they are rarely thought by the medical establishment to be doing so. Sam and the sound technician are just two of the nearly 12 million people in the U.S. who have been treated for cancer and are able to wait watchfully in large part due to the incremental success of cancer treatments.[2] And there are others: people who have had heart attacks who are at increased risk for another and people with HIV whose viral load will likely one day cross the threshold to full-blown AIDS.[3,4]

The event we await is not a certainty for any of us. Many of us live long and well with each of these conditions and diseases. Some of us die of different causes altogether. But the current of anxiety about what is to come runs through our days, sometimes palpable, sometime deep below the surface.

So what? Everyone's going to die of something sometime. Any one of us could be hit by a bus tomorrow. Well, yes. But watchful waiting post-cancer or post-HIV diagnosis or post-heart attack means that a bus with my name on it may be headed straight at me and it is not clear if I am going to be able to leap out of the way. This makes us vigilant, slightly on edge, even when there is no bus in view.

What can we learn from observing or being part of this growing number of waiters?

For one thing, people respond to such uncertainty in very different ways. Some shut it out: If it happens, it happens. We have been sufficiently imposed upon by the experience of this disease or illness to date and prefer to "jump off the (next) bridge when we come to it." We tend not to participate in monitoring and testing. Some people slowly get used to the uncertainty over time; the distress that accompanies the testing and any new symptom (like the fear that a headache might be a brain tumor) subsides. We construct a new life around the limitations imposed by the condition and carry on, despite occasional flurries of anxiety and the occasional sleepless night.[5]

Some of us find the idea of waiting in the face of an impending threat too passive a strategy, and we take matters into our own hands. We insist on surgery or medication now or we demand more frequent testing. We devise our own dietary, physical and mental regimens and employ a range of alternative medicine approaches in an effort to reduce the risk we face and reclaim some sense that we can control our future.[6-9]

The manner in which we watchfully wait may shift as the meaning of our illness and its threat changes over time. Despite our varied responses, however, we share more than just an undercurrent of anxiety.

Each of us has glimpsed the limits of science and medicine. As people who are by definition seeking to be made whole again through medical intervention, this is particularly sobering.

Most of us have had some experience with finding and using health care services by the time we arrive at a point of watchful waiting. This means that we might know more about how to obtain services, but it is no guarantee that we are wiser about making good use of them, nor does it mean that we are more prepared to wait.

And every single one of us wishes that bus didn't have our name on it.

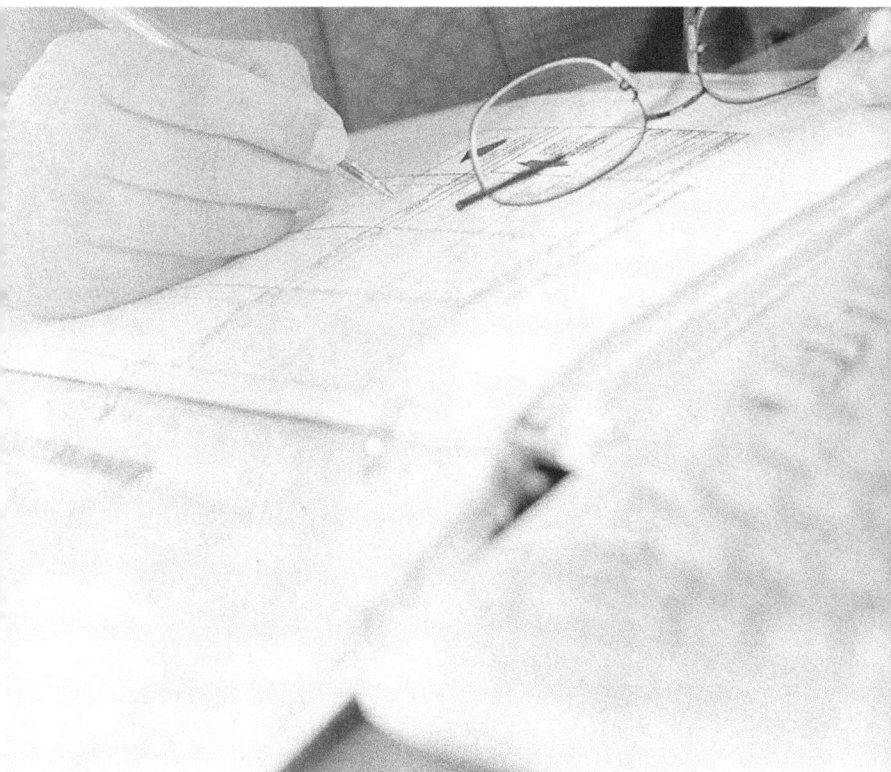

11

Poster Child for Survivorship Planning

am a poster child for why everyone who has had cancer needs to work with his or her doctor(s) to develop and implement a survivorship plan.

Two of my four cancer-related diagnoses were found during routine screenings. Two of my cancer-related diagnoses and one serious heart condition were probably due to late effects of cancer treatment when I was young.

Each was a complete surprise to me, and while there is evidence that predicts most of these occurrences, not one of my doctors used this literature to shape a plan for my post-treatment care.

I was on my own. My fear of yet another recurrence led me over time to cobble together a motley collection of oncologists (one for each body part) and other specialists (cardiologist, dermatologist, endocrinologist, and so forth) to watch over me. I thought I was lucky that this has worked so far.

But since I became a patient at Memorial Sloan-Kettering's Adult Long-Term Follow-Up Program two years ago and I now have a formal survivorship plan, I *know* I was lucky. The success of my haphazard plan was most likely due to its "even a stopped clock is right twice a day" approach — an extraordinarily bad use of time and resources, mine and my insurer's. Now that I am working with a knowledgeable physician, I can see how rudimentary and inadequate my efforts were.[1]

Anyone who has experienced (or witnessed) the impact of a cancer diagnosis and the disruption — physical, emotional, social — of treatment knows that the experience of cancer doesn't end with that final appointment in the chemotherapy suite.

I am not alone in my lack of a survivorship plan. Most people who complete the initial intense part of treatment for cancer do not have a formal plan for their ongoing care once that phase is over. The aim of care after active treatment is to return the person to health and functioning, prevent a recurrence or detect it early, minimize long-term side effects and treat conditions that result from the toxic effects of chemotherapy, surgery or radiation.[2]

Raising the priority and value of (and insurance coverage for) survivorship care has been the focus of the Office of Cancer Survivorship at the National Cancer Institute, which funds research on the long-term effects of treatment, and is supported by CDC's Cancer Survivorship efforts to implement those findings.[3,4] The National Coalition for Cancer Survivorship has worked with the Institute of Medicine's National Cancer Policy Forum and Congress to define what constitutes survivorship care and eliminate the barriers to its delivery.[5,6] The American Society of Clinical Oncology has implemented standards for treatment summaries for survivorship care.[7]

Nevertheless, progress toward implementing a personalized survivorship plan for each person treated for cancer in the U.S. seems stalled. There are many reasons for this, most related to the organization and incentives of health care delivery, the knowledge, interest and proclivities of various health professionals, and the twin demands of cost control and evidence-based care.

Where does this leave those of us who have completed the first intensive phase of cancer treatment?

Mostly on our own, looking for a knowledgeable oncologist or primary care clinician who is willing to stay on top of the emerging evidence to help us match our risks and needs to the tests and services that will keep us as healthy as possible.

I recently gave a talk at a meeting sponsored by the National Cancer Institute that spells out in detail what we patients (and our loved ones) currently have to do to develop and implement a good, solid survivorship care plan.

I concluded that I have learned two lessons about survivorship from my experiences as a person living with cancer:

First, regardless of the excellence of the data, the promise of reimbursement and the skill of the physician, if I don't show up, discuss my risks and my options and then follow through on the decisions I make with my clinician, I will get no benefit from survivorship planning, nor from the tests and technologies that can be used to improve the quality and extend the length of my life. These are the things that only I, with help from my caregivers, can do.

And second, I know with complete certainty that regardless of how much expertise, experience and energy I invest in developing and implementing a survivorship plan, I cannot do this alone.

An effective survivorship plan requires an active partnership between the patient and his or her provider.

12

Lessons from the Year of Living Sickishly

"**B**uck up. You are going to feel bad for a year."

This was my chemotherapy nurse a year ago, returning a call I made to my oncologist. I had left a message asking whether there was something he could do to help me. Should I feel this horrible following three action-packed months that included stomach cancer surgery and aggressive chemotherapy?

The answer, at least as far as my nurse was concerned, was "Yes."

And she was right. It did take a year to regain my energy and feel well again.

The new year set me reflecting upon what I've learned about being sick over the past 12 months that only the experience itself could teach me:

You know that old Supremes song, "You Can't Hurry Love"? I learned that you can't necessarily hurry healing either, even if you work hard at it. A week after that call to my oncologist — still feeling rocky — I joined a local gym's "$30 for 30 days" New Year's special to try to revive my cardiovascular fitness. For each of the next 30 days, I trudged down there, got on that Nordic Track machine and forced myself to flail about for 40 laborious minutes. On most days last year, I made myself walk at least a mile and practice yoga. I did my level best to choke down a tiny healthy snack almost every waking hour. Often, doing these simple tasks took all the energy and will I possessed. But I was committed, convinced that if I did them I would get better faster.

And it still took a year before I felt normal again. How frustrating was that?

I have absorbed the very American notion that success results from hard work. By extension, health should be achievable if we comply with the admonitions of our employers, the media and health promotion advocates to exercise and eat right. I knew that my behavior didn't cause my cancer and wasn't going to cure it. But surely, I thought, I can speed up my recovery from the assault of chemotherapy and surgery if I really try. I had great expectations. So did those around me: "Why is she still so frail?" "Why isn't she better yet?"

I might still be feeling pokey if I hadn't worked so hard at recovering. But this experience slammed me up against the reality of physical illness and the limits of behavior in changing its course. It reminded me how a deep belief in our own efficacy makes it easy to slip into blaming ourselves (or the sick person) for not getting better. And it reminded me of how unruly, unpredictable and often uncontrollable the effects of disease and its treatment are on our bodies.

Another lesson: I expected that health information technology (HIT) advances and opportunities to connect with other patients using social media would dramatically change my experience of treatment in contrast to my previous three experiences with cancer.

This time around, I was dazzled by the ease with which I was able to collect the information and evidence I needed to make good decisions about my treatment plan. And I am grateful for online access to friends and colleagues all over the world that allowed me to feel less isolated over this past year than I have during previous illnesses.

But once I started treatment, feeling ill extinguished my curiosity about my disease. It dampened all interest in second-guessing treatment decisions or seeking innovative approaches or learning about new technologies to aid my recovery. And only occasionally could I summon the energy to reach out even to close friends and family, much less to seek out people like me online for advice and support.

I see embedded in the enthusiasm about patient portals, decision aids and smartphones an attitude that being actively engaged with new technologies can somehow provide happy relief from the pain and discomfort of illness.[1-5] Bright health information websites, fun games designed to inspire adherence and smart medication reminder apps are presented as having the potential to turn the experience of illness into a series of problems that are easily solved through the acquisition of technologies.[6-9]

It's true that HIT can help with scheduling appointments, refilling prescriptions and coordinating the disposition of test results to different clinicians, for example. (My clinicians mostly don't use electronic health records with patient portals, so I had no respite from those tasks.) And remote patient monitoring and assistive devices already make some caregiving chores easier. These are welcome contributions, especially as more responsibilities for care are shifted to patients and their families. But I return to the world of the healthy with the impression that the value of HIT is tactical, not transformative, at least for the sick person: There is no app for suffering.

My third insight from the past year is that most of the time I believed I was thinking clearly, but in hindsight, I see that my judgment and thought processes were often clouded. Through my experience with serious illnesses, I've developed strategies for getting through the days. For example, regardless of how I feel, I always bathe, dress, eat breakfast and put my shoes on. The shoes are important: They serve as an optimistic signal to me that I'm well enough to get up and go outside just like anyone else. Between the shoes and my exercise and diet routine, I could sometimes convince myself that I had returned to my former healthy state (conveniently forgetting my need to lie on the couch for hours).

But I had not recovered, and the clarity of my thinking was often, although not consistently, compromised. I scheduled events and travel that were unrealistic given my stamina, and when I couldn't be dissuaded from following through, I'd spend days recuperating. Again and again I disappointed myself and others by setting ambitious goals for commitments I wasn't ready to meet.

I know I am not unique in this. I watch friends and colleagues whose judgment is impaired by illness make similar, often higher-stakes errors. They make weird self-care choices, abruptly change treatment decisions, impulsively fire their physicians and refuse to seek advice about clearly serious conditions. We all believe that we are making rational choices when we do these things. But we aren't, and the effect on our health and recovery can be serious.

I wanted to write about these three insights while they are still vivid for me. Standing for the past couple of months on the shifting border between illness and health, I've experienced how (fortunately) easy it is to forget how illness eats away at the balance of one's mind, body and spirit. As a mostly ill person glancing into the world of the healthy over the past year, I've marveled at the insensitivity and indifference to this imbalance by even those with the greatest love, or best intentions, training and experience.

The tools, technologies and services that constitute health care will never completely eliminate the suffering caused by illness, even if they are perfectly delivered. But that suffering might take a more modest toll if all of us — patients, professionals, caregivers, family, friends and colleagues — have clearer expectations about the arc of illness and how it affects and can be affected by each of us.

In the end, that curt directive by my chemotherapy nurse to "Buck up. You are going to feel bad for a year" was the most helpful advice I received.

References

"Patient Engagement!" Our Skin Is in the Game

1. Judith Hibbard profile. University of Oregon. Last Revised February 4, 2013. http://pages.uoregon.edu/jhibbard/

2. Patient Activation Measure. Insignia Health. http://www.insigniahealth.com/solutions/patient-activation-measure

3. Kate Lorig profile. Stanford School of Medicine. http://patienteducation.stanford.edu/staff.html

4. Chronic Disease Self-Management Program. Stanford School of Medicine. http://patienteducation.stanford.edu/programs/cdsmp.html

5. Victor Montori profile. Mayo Clinic. http://mayoresearch.mayo.edu/staff/montori_vm.cfm

6. Noncompliance –Victor Montori, M.D. You Tube. http://www.youtube.com/watch?v=flcRKdoaiVk

7. David Sobel profile. Kaiser Permanente. http://xnet.kp.org/kpinternational/faculty/sobel.html

8. Prepared Patient Blog. Posts by author David Sobel. http://www.cfah.org/blog/posts-by-author/David-Sobel

9. The Smokers' Surcharge. The New York Times. November, 16, 2011. http://www.nytimes.com/2011/11/17/health/policy/smokers-penalized-with-health-insurance-premiums.html?_r=3&ref=business&

Another Devastating Diagnosis to Face

1. Aftershock: What to Do When the Doctor Gives You—or Someone You Love—a Devastating Diagnosis. Jessie Gruman. Walker Publishing, second edition, 2010. http://www.aftershockbook.com/

Contemplating Safety While Lying Down

1. To Err Is Human: Building a Safer Health System. National Academy of Sciences. 2000. http://www.nap.edu/catalog.php?record_id=9728

2. Susan E. Sheridan profile. Consumers Advancing Patient Safety. http://www.patientsafety.org/page/94909/

3. Consumers Advancing Patient Safety. http://www.patientsafety.org/page/home/;jsessionid=g2erjf62inmx

4. National Patient Safety Foundation. http://www.npsf.org/

5. Hospital Performance Reports: Impact on Quality, Market Share, and Reputation. Health Affairs. July 2005. http://content.healthaffairs.org/content/24/4/1150.abstract

Hospital Discharge Without a Net

1. Hospital Readmissions Reduction Program. http://www.bricker.com/documents/resources/reform/reformbill42.pdf

2. Hospital Compare. Medicare.gov. http://www.medicare.gov/hospitalcompare/

3. Hospitals Work to Reduce Wait Times, Readmission Rates. Kaiser Health News. July 18, 2010. http://www.kaiserhealthnews.org/daily-reports/2010/june/18/readmits-and-wait-times.aspx

4. Health Reform Takes Aim at Hospital Readmissions Rates. U.S. News & World Report. July 21, 2010. http://health.usnews.com/health-news/best-hospitals/articles/2010/07/21/health-reform-takes-aim-at-hospital-readmission-rates

5. Rehospitalizations among Patients in the Medicare Fee-for-Service Program. NEJM. 2009. http://www.nejm.org/doi/full/10.1056/NEJMsa0803563?siteid=nejm&ijkey=3COjS3yxXjOtYkeytype%3Dref&&

6. World Congress. http://www.worldcongress.com/

7. Institute for Healthcare Improvement. http://www.ihi.org/offerings/Pages/default.aspx

8. Why Ask if You Won't Help Me. Prepared Patient blog. July 28, 2010. http://www.cfah.org/blog/2010/why-ask-if-you-wont-help-me

9. Federal Patient Self-Determination Act Final Regulations. http://www.cobar.org/docs/psda.pdf?ID=1816

10. OBRA '90 at Sweet Sixteen: A Retrospective Review. U.S. Pharmacist. 2008. http://www.uspharmacist.com/content/d/featured_articles/c/10126/

11. Centers for Medicare & Medicaid Services, HHS. http://1.usa.gov/174n4Uy

12. Patient, Heal Thyself. The Wall Street Journal. October 25, 2010. http://online.wsj.com/article/SB10001424052702304248704575574172720039534.html

13. Eric A. Coleman bio. Care Transitions Intervention. http://www.innovativecaremodels.com/care_models/12/leaders

14. Transitional Care Model. http://www.transitionalcare.info/

15. Project Red. Boston University. http://www.bu.edu/fammed/projectred/meetlouise.html

A Valentine to Shared Decision Making

1. Society for Medical Decision Making. http://www.smdm.org/

2. Patient Decision Aids. Ottawa Hospital Research Institute. May 7, 2013. http://decisionaid.ohri.ca/index.html

3. The World Congress 3rd Annual Leadership Summit on Shared Decision Making. September 19-20, 2013. http://www.worldcongress.com/events/HL13011/

4. Shared Decision Making About Screening and Chemoprevention. U.S. Preventive Services Task Force. http://bit.ly/14yOLTn

5. Informed Medical Decisions Foundation. http://informedmedicaldecisions.org/

One Small Step for Patient-Centered Care, One Less Barrier to Engagement

1. Patient-Centered Primary Care Collaborative. http://www.pcpcc.net/about

2. Consumer Health Digest. http://www.consumerhealthdigest.com/

3. The "Meaningful Use" Regulation for Electronic Health Records. NEJM. August 5, 2010. http://www.nejm.org/doi/full/10.1056/NEJMp1006114

4. Creating a Patient Guide for a Clinic or Medical Practice. Center for Advancing Health. 2011. http://www.cfah.org/engagement/research/creating-a-patient-guide-for-a-clinic-or-medical-practice

I am not My iPhone

1. You Love Your iPhone. Literally. The New York Times. The Opinion Pages. September 20, 2011. http://www.nytimes.com/2011/10/01/opinion/you-love-your-iphone-literally.html?_r=0

2. The iPhone and the Brain. The New York Times. The Opinion Pages. October 4, 2011. http://www.nytimes.com/2011/10/05/opinion/the-iphone-and-the-brain.html?_r=2&ref=todayspaper&

3. Is Mobile Health the Next Killer App? NYC Health Business Leaders. October 12, 2011. http://mobilehealthnychbl.eventbrite.com/

4. Groups Tap Funding for Mobile Health Efforts Targeting Seniors With Chronic Conditions. iHealthBeat. September 22, 2011. http://mobilehealthnychbl.eventbrite.com/

5. Is Mobile the Prescription for Sustained Behavior Change? Health Innoventions. September 27, 2011. http://www.healthinnoventions.org/wp-content/uploads/downloads/2011/09/Is-Mobile-the-Prescription-for-Sustained-Behavior-Change_Health-Innoventions_Models-for-Change_Oct-12-13-2011.pdf

The Lemon of Illness and the Demand for Lemonade

1. As You Like It. Shakespeare. The Tech.
   http://shakespeare.mit.edu/asyoulikeit/full.html

2. Experimental Research on Just-World Theory: Problems, Developments, and Future Challenges. Psychological Bulletin. 2005.
   http://www.brocku.ca/psychology/people/Hafer_Begue_05.pdf

3. A Reader in the Anthropology of Religion. 2002.
   http://www.amazon.com/Reader-Anthropology-Religion-Michael-Lambek/dp/1405136146

4. Columbia University Medical Center Program in Narrative Medicine. Faculty Publications.
   http://narrativemedicine.org/bibliography.html

5. Reference List of Writing/Disclosure Studies. April 2013.
   http://homepage.psy.utexas.edu/HomePage/Faculty/Pennebaker/Reprints/writingrefs.htm

6. A meta-analytic review of benefit finding and growth. Journal of Consulting and Clinical Psychology. October 2006.
   http://psycnet.apa.org/journals/ccp/74/5/797/

Appointment in Samarra: Our Lives of Watchful Waiting

1. Prepared Patient: Watchful Waiting: When Treatment Can Wait.
   http://www.cfah.org/prepared-patient/prepared-patient-articles/watchful-waiting-when-treatment-can-wait

2. US cancer survivors grows to nearly 12 million. National Cancer Institute. March 10, 2011. http://www.cancer.gov/newscenter/newsfromnci/2011/survivorshipMMWR2011

3. AHA Statistical Update. Circulation. 2011. http://circ.ahajournals.org/content/123/4/e18.full

4. Changing Patterns of HIV Epidemiology, United States 2011. CDC.
   http://www.acthiv.org/2011_presentations/opening_plenary_040711/John%20T.%20Brooks.pdf

5. Watchful waiting. Just eat your cupcake blog. April 16, 2011.
   http://www.acthiv.org/2011_presentations/opening_plenary_040711/John%20T.%20Brooks.pdf

6. Diet May Cut Risk of Cancer Recurring. The Washington Post. May 17, 2005. http://www.washingtonpost.com/wp-dyn/content/article/2005/05/16/AR2005051600353.html

7. Exercise and HIV. Aidsinfonet.org. February 28, 2013.
   http://www.aidsinfonet.org/fact_sheets/view/802

8. Meditation and cancer patients. ABC News. March 21, 2011 http://abclocal.go.com/wabc/story?section=news/health&id=8025122

9. Heart Disease: Alternative Medicine. Mayo Clinic. January 16, 2013. http://www.mayoclinic.com/health/heart-disease/DS01120/DSECTION=alternative-medicine

Poster Child for Survivorship Planning

1. Kevin C. Oeffinger profile. Memorial Sloan-Kettering Cancer Center. http://www.mskcc.org/cancer-care/doctor/kevin-oeffinger

2. A National Action Plan for Cancer Survivorship: Advancing Public Health Strategies. Center for Disease Control and Prevention. April 2004. http://www.cdc.gov/cancer/survivorship/pdf/plan.pdf

3. Cancer Survivorship Research. National Cancer Institute. October 16, 2012. http://dccps.nci.nih.gov/ocs/about.html

4. What CDC Is Doing About Cancer Survivorship. Center for Disease Control and Prevention. January 16, 2013. http://1.usa.gov/ZKUGBn

5. National Coalition for Cancer Survivorship. http://www.canceradvocacy.org/

6. National Cancer Policy Forum. Institute of Medicine. March 29, 2013. http://www.canceradvocacy.org/

7. ASCO Cancer Treatment Summaries. Cancer.net. March 13, 2013. http://www.cancer.net/survivorship/asco-cancer-treatment-summaries

Lessons from the Year of Living Sickishly

1. Patient Portal. Chart Logic. http://www.chartlogic.com/patient-portal/

2. EMR: The Patient Portal. PrognoCIS. http://www.emrexperts.com/articles/emr-patient-portal.php

3. Our Approach: Collaborative Medical Decision Making. Expert Medical Navigation. March 15, 2011. http://www.exmednav.com/2011/03/15/our-approach-collaborative-medical-decision-making/

4. Weighty Choices, in Patients' Hands. The Wall Street Journal. August 4, 2009. http://online.wsj.com/article/SB10001424052970203674704574328570637446770.html

5. As Smartphones Get Smarter, You May Get Healthier: How mHealth Can Bring Cheaper Health Care to All. Fast Company. February 2012. http://www.fastcompany.com/1802735/smartphones-get-smarter-you-may-get-healthier-how-mhealth-can-bring-cheaper-health-care-all

6. Games for Global Health. http://gamesforhealth.org/

7. Discovery fit and Health. http://health.discovery.com/

8. MedCenter 4 Alarm Talking Reminder Clock-Med Center. http://www.amazon.com/Medcenter-Talking-Alarm-Medication-Reminder/dp/B000VUM79G

9. MyMedSchedule.com http://www.mymedschedule.com/

Jessie Gruman

Jessie Gruman is president and founder of the Center for Advancing Health, a nonpartisan, Washington-based policy institute which, since 1992, has been supported by foundations and individuals to work on people's engagement in their health care from the patient perspective. Dr. Gruman draws on her own experience of treatment for four cancer diagnoses, interviews with patients and caregivers, surveys and peer-reviewed research as the basis of her work to describe and advocate for policies and practices to overcome the challenges people face in finding good care and getting the most from it.

Dr. Gruman has worked on this same set of concerns in the private sector (AT&T), the public sector (National Cancer Institute) and the voluntary health sector (American Cancer Society). She holds a B.A. from Vassar College and a Ph.D. in Social Psychology from Columbia University and is a Professorial Lecturer in the School of Public Health and Health Services at the George Washington University. She currently serves on the boards of the Center for Medical Technology Policy, VillageCare in New York City and the Sallan Foundation.

Dr. Gruman has received honorary doctorates from Brown University, Carnegie Mellon University, Clark University, Georgetown University, New York University, Northeastern University, Salve Regina University, Syracuse University and Tulane University, and the Presidential Medal of the George Washington University. She was honored by Research!America for her leadership in advocacy for health research, is a fellow of the Society for Behavioral Medicine and the New York Academy of Medicine and a member of the American Academy of Arts and Sciences and the Council on Foreign Relations.

Dr. Gruman is the author of *AfterShock: What to Do When the Doctor Gives You – or Someone You Love – a Devastating Diagnosis* (Walker Publishing, second edition, 2010); *The Experience of the American Patient: Risk, Trust and Choice* (Health Behavior Media, 2009); *Behavior Matters* (Health Behavior Media, 2008) as well as scientific papers, opinion essays and articles. She blogs regularly on the Prepared Patient Blog at cfah.org/blog and tweets daily @jessiegruman.